Ketogenic Diet Desserts

Quick and Easy Low Carb Keto Diet Recipes

Madison Miller

Copyrights

Disclaimer and Terms of Use

ISBN: 978-1539530046

Printed in the United States

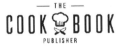

— THE —
COOK BOOK
PUBLISHER

Avant-Propos

If you have been a ketogenic lifestyle, then you understand the incredible benefits of doing so – from weight loss to increased energy and overall improved health. But did you know that the ketogenic diet is also one of the few dietary lifestyles that allows you to eat sweet, decadent desserts without a hint of guilt? So many of the keto-friendly foods that are already in your kitchen can be used to create some of the most delicious and satisfying desserts, with the help of the recipes in this book. With a focus on natural, unprocessed foods, it becomes possible to enjoy the sweet treats you crave while adhering to the lifestyle that is so important to you. With recipes for everything from creamy ice creams to irresistible cookies, this collection of keto-friendly dessert recipes will not sabotage your diet or leave a single sweet craving unsatisfied.

Contents

Introduction

There are some things in this world that are simply too sweet to resist. You work hard, you make your health a priority, so why shouldn't you be able to reward yourself with the sweet decadence of a perfect dessert? Sweet treats have been the recipient of a bad reputation, and to be honest some of them deserve it, especially the ones that are loaded with bad fats and processed ingredients. And there are people, just like you, who have committed to following a specific dietary lifestyle and have decided that most desserts are just off the table as options. If you are feeling that your ketogenic diet has limited your opportunities for satisfying your sweet tooth, then the time has come to change your thinking and open your mind. There are literally hundreds of keto approved desserts, and this book highlights some of the best.

What is the image in your mind of the perfect dessert? I think this answer would be different depending upon whom you asked. Some people like the sweet simplicity of lightly enhanced fruit desserts, while others choose to go all in for rich, sweet decadence, and there is a whole spectrum in between. In this book, we have strived to provide a little of everything and show you just how easy it can be to have your dessert, no matter what the perfect dessert is for you. You are about to experience a collection of cookies, pies, and elegant desserts that are suitable for any occasion. We have also included decadent keto bombs and amazing mug cakes that are perfect for when you just want a quick, sweet nibble.

We all know that the key to staying on track for any diet is keeping it simple, and also keeping it realistic. When you feel deprived in any way, you are more likely to stray off of your intended nutritional path. One of the main culprits of diet sabotage is without question dessert. Who wants to live a life devoid of a little sweetness? You might have chosen the ketogenic lifestyle because a doctor or nutritionist recommended it to you because of a preexisting condition or dietary needs. Maybe you are a devout low carb eater and prefer the ketogenic ratios, or perhaps low carb, ketogenic eating is entirely new to you but you are loving the results and want to make it a long term commitment. It really doesn't matter how or why you came to the keto diet, the desserts in this book are suitable for you no matter what your keto beginnings.

So, take the recipes in this book and embrace the sweeter side of the ketogenic life.

A Note Regarding Frozen Ice Cream Recipes

The ice cream recipes in this book were designed to use an ice cream maker. If you are lucky enough to have one of these, just follow the instructions included with your device when creating the frozen recipes in this book. If you do not have an ice cream maker, you can still enjoy these recipes; it just takes a little bit more work.

When making ice cream without an ice cream maker, first combine all the ingredients together as directed, except for any solid add-ins such as nuts, coconut, or chunks of fruit.

Next, place the liquid in a shallow container, such as a baking dish, and put it in the freezer. Every thirty to forty minutes, remove the container from the freezer and stir.

Once the liquid begins to thicken, but is still thin enough to stir with a spoon, you can then put in the solid additions. Adding them at this point prevents them from immediately settling on the bottom of the pan.

At some point, the ice cream will become too thick to stir with a spoon. When that happens you can scrape it with either a fork or an ice cream scoop.

When your ice cream is almost completely frozen, you can then place it in a blender or food processor and give it a quick whirl. You can also use an immersion blender if you have one. This step provides a creamier consistency to the finished product.

Finally, place the ice cream back in the freezer and let it harden to the desired consistency before enjoying it.

The Making of a Ketogenic Dessert: The Haves and the Have Nots

Many people think that eating low carb for any amount of time is either too complicated or too boring. Luckily, you and I both know better. All you need to enjoy delicious keto desserts is a solid understanding of what keto-approved foods can be crafted into desserts and the knowledge of how to put them together. Once you have that, your dessert creations will not be confined to those you find in this book, or any other, for that matter. Putting together keto desserts is actually quite simple. Rich creamy foods are perfect for desserts, and just a touch of sweet brings out their decadence. Here is a list of dessert foods that are a big no (you likely already know these) and a list of foods you can embrace (some of which might surprise you). Take a good look and then prepare your grocery list – because for you, dessert is back on the menu.

The Haves

Many of the foods you enjoy in your typical keto meals and snacks can be used to create sweet treats as well. Here in this book you will see some of the same ingredients repeatedly used. This is for two reasons. First of all, it makes it easier on your pantry and your wallet and secondly, some keto-friendly ingredients just naturally lend themselves to creamy, sweet goodness without many alterations or additives. Here is a list of what you are going to want to have on hand to create a great keto dessert anytime.

Sweeteners: You are eating the ketogenic way, which means your health is important to you. You likely care about the quality and integrity of the ingredients you use, and understand that the more natural they are, the better. For this reason we try to stay away from artificial sweeteners in favor of low carbohydrate, low calorie natural alternatives. The two you will see most often in this book are erythritol, which is a natural sugar alcohol that is available in granulated or powdered forms, and stevia, which is plant-derived and available in liquid or powder forms. If your carbohydrate limit is a little higher, you can also use small amounts of pure maple syrup, honey, or molasses.

The Creamy Stuff: One of the things to love the most about the ketogenic diet is how it favors rich, creamy ingredients. It turns out that these are also great for creating decadent desserts. The important thing to remember is that a ketogenic diet depends on a high fat, low sugar ratio, so make sure you are always choosing full fat dairy products and products that do not contain any hidden sweeteners. For the recipes in this book, use rich and creamy ingredients – such as heavy whipping cream, full fat sour cream, full fat cream cheese, whole unflavored yogurt, mascarpone cheese, whole ricotta cheese, whole cream butter, unsweetened full fat coconut milk and coconut cream (the cream that rises to the top of pure coconut milk when it is refrigerated).

Nuts: One of the best ways to add fat, protein, and fiber, not to mention flavor, is by using a variety of nuts in your desserts. They are great additives that provide texture and character to dessert dishes. Make sure that the nuts you choose are not pre-seasoned with anything sweet. Depending on your other dietary restrictions and preferences you might prefer to go for raw and unsalted. Almonds and walnuts are the best ketogenic choices. However, cashews, pecans, peanuts, and pistachios are also great options as long as you don't overindulge. Remember that nuts can also raise your calorie intake rather quickly. For most people who choose to eat the ketogenic way, this is not a problem since the general idea is the more calories the merrier, however if you are calorie restricted, pay close attention to the portion sizes of nuts.

Eggs: There really isn't much that needs to be said about this keto perfect food. They are rich in protein, provide the right kind of fats, and are essential in many dishes both sweet and savory. Keep plenty of these guys on hand.

Fruits: You might think that if you are choosing to eat low carb that you are choosing to forgo all fruit. This simply isn't true. There are many fruits that can be enjoyed, in limited quantities, on the ketogenic diet. The best fruits for ketogenic eating are berries, including blueberries, blackberries, raspberries, and strawberries. If you are fortunate enough to live where you have access to other wild berries such as huckleberries or logan berries, then by all means, include them too. Berries are relatively low in carbs, offer healthy antioxidants and are sweet, juicy little nuggets that quickly satisfy sweet cravings. Additionally, other fruits can be used in small amounts. These include avocados, coconut, cantaloupe, watermelon, lemons, limes, plums, and peaches.

The Have Nots

Sweeteners: It is hard to think of enjoying a dessert without the addition of a sweetener. As you already know, there are natural options for sweetening your food and drinks without using actual sugar. Sugar is loaded with carbohydrates and promotes inflammation in the body. You should avoid pure white sugar, brown sugar, powdered sugar and artificial sweeteners, unless otherwise suggested by your physician. Natural alternatives such as honey or molasses can be used in scant amounts depending upon your daily carbohydrate intake level.

Grains: When preparing your keto desserts, you will want to stay away from traditional grain based flours and other grains such as oats, barley, etc. Nut flours are an excellent alternative and take little or no adaptations to substitute into a recipe.

Dairy: When eating the ketogenic way, cheese and cream are among the things that you can enjoy. Their lesser fat counterparts, however are not. Stay away from low fat milk, skim milk cheeses and low fat yogurts, especially those with artificial sweeteners.

Fruits: For the most part, you will want to stick to berries and small amounts of the additional fruits that we have listed above. Fruits that have high sugar saturation, such as tropical fruits should be avoided, unless consumed in very small amounts with adequate fat and protein to balance them out. For instance, you cannot eat half a mango, but you can have a little mango that has been pureed into a creamy popsicle base.

Diet Sodas and other artificially flavored beverages: Sometimes all you need to calm a raging sweet tooth is a nice, cold sweet drink. Diet sodas do not contain real sugars, so you would think that they would be fine to drink any time. However, it appears that diet beverages contribute to increased sweet cravings and some people have reported going out of ketosis when drinking too many of them. If you must have your diet soda, do so sparingly and save them for special occasions.

Fruity and Decadent

Blackberry Pavlovas

Serves: 6

Ingredients
4 egg whites
½ cup erythritol
½ teaspoon hazelnut extract
1 teaspoon vanilla extract
1 teaspoon lemon juice
2 teaspoons xanthan gum
1 cup heavy cream
1 cup blackberries
1 teaspoon lemon zest
½ cup almonds, slivered

Directions
1. Preheat the oven to 300°F and line a baking sheet with parchment paper.
2. Using a pencil, trace six circles on the parchment paper, each measuring approximately five inches in diameter.
3. Place the egg whites in a bowl and beat on medium-high speed until they are thick and foamy.
4. Still using the electric mixer, add the erythritol in two to three increments, mixing until stiff peaks form.
5. Add in the hazelnut extract, vanilla extract, lemon juice, and xanthan gum. Gently fold them in with a rubber spatula, until just mixed.
6. Spoon the mixture out onto the baking sheet, using the traced circles as a guide. Using the back of a spoon, press an indent in the center of each mound.
7. Place the baking sheet in the oven and bake for 50-55 minutes, or until golden.

8. While the shells are baking, combine the heavy cream, blackberries, and lemon zest in a blender. Blend until smooth and thickened.
9. Place the mixture in the refrigerator and chill until the shells are baked.
10. Remove the shells from the oven and allow them to cool enough to handle.
11. Spoon the blackberry mixture into the center of each shell.
12. Garnish with sliced almonds before serving.

Nutritional Information
Calories 206.2, Total Fat 18.8 g,
Total Carbs 6.0 g, Approx. Net Carbs 3.8 g, Dietary Fiber 2.2 g,
Sugars 2.2 g, Protein 5.1 g

Triple Berry Cheesecake in a Mug

Serves: 4

Ingredients:
¼ cup butter
½ cup almond flour
1 tablespoon erythritol
1 cup cream cheese
½ cup heavy cream
¼ cup sour cream
1 vanilla bean, scraped
1 teaspoon lemon zest
2 teaspoons lemon juice
¼ cup blackberries
¼ cup raspberries
¼ cup blueberries
1 tablespoon water

Directions:
1. Melt the butter in a saucepan over medium heat.
2. Add the almond flour and erythritol. Cook, stirring frequently, for 1-2 minutes. Remove the pot from the heat and set it aside.
3. In a bowl, combine the cream cheese, heavy cream, sour cream, vanilla, lemon zest, and lemon juice.
4. Using an electric mixer, blend until the mixture is thick and creamy. Cover and chill for 15 minutes.
5. In a separate saucepan, combine the blackberries, raspberries, blueberries, and water. Add a little more erythritol if you prefer your berries to be more sweet.
6. Cook over medium-low heat, stirring frequently, just until the berries begin to break down. Remove them from the heat.

7. Spoon the cream mixture into 4 serving mugs.
8. Top with the berry mixture and a sprinkling of the almond flour crumble before serving.

Nutritional Information
Calories 527.3, Total Fat 52.6 g,
Total Carbs 10.1 g, Approx. Net Carbs 7.4 g, Dietary Fiber 2.7 g,
Sugars 4.0 g, Protein 8.7 g

Blueberry Buckle Pudding Pots

Serves: 4

Ingredients:
½ cup coconut flour
½ teaspoon baking powder
10 egg yolks
½ cup butter
1 tablespoon heavy cream
1 tablespoon lemon juice
¼ cup erythritol
20 drops liquid stevia
1 teaspoon cinnamon
1 tablespoon fresh ground ginger
1 cup blueberries

Directions:
1. Preheat the oven to 350°F and lightly oil 4 ramekins.
2. In a bowl, combine the coconut flour and baking powder. Mix and set aside.
3. Beat the egg yolks in a separate bowl until they are light yellow and frothy.
4. Add the butter, heavy cream, and lemon juice to the egg yolks. Blend until smooth.
5. Next, add the erythritol, stevia, cinnamon, and ginger. Mix well.
6. Add the dry ingredients into the wet and mix just until combined.
7. Fold in the blueberries.
8. Spoon the mixture into the ramekins and place them in the oven.
9. Bake for 25 minutes or until firm set.
10. Remove them from the oven and allow them to cool slightly before serving.

Nutritional Information

Calories 436.6, Total Fat 37.1 g,
Total Carbs 15.7 g, Approx. Net Carbs 6.7 g, Dietary Fiber 9.0 g,
Sugars 5.0 g, Protein 10.8 g

Spiced Orange Pots De Crème

Serves: 4

Ingredients:
4 egg yolks
¼ cup powdered erythritol
¼ cup blood orange juice
1 ½ cups heavy cream
20 drops liquid stevia
¼ teaspoon salt
½ teaspoon cinnamon
½ teaspoon ground clove
1 tablespoon orange zest
1 teaspoon vanilla extract
1 teaspoon maple syrup extract
¼ teaspoon xanthan gum

Directions:
1. Preheat the oven to 300°F.
2. Place the egg yolks in a bowl and mix until creamy. Set them aside.
3. Combine the powdered erythritol and blood orange juice together in a small saucepan.
4. In another saucepan, combine the heavy cream, liquid stevia, salt, cinnamon, clove, orange zest, and vanilla extract.
5. Place both saucepans on the stovetop and bring them to a boil over medium to medium-high heat.
6. Once the cream mixture begins to boil, reduce the heat to low and whisk well. Stir occasionally as the sauce continues to cook for 3-5 more minutes.
7. Once the blood orange mixture begins to boil, add the maple syrup extract and the xanthan gum. Reduce the heat to low and simmer until the liquid begins to thicken.

8. Remove both saucepans from the heat and add the syrup mixture into the cream mixture.
9. Take several tablespoons of the warm sauce and slowly add it to the egg yolks. Whisk well while adding, to temper the eggs and prevent them from scrambling as you add the rest of the sauce.
10. Add the remaining cream to the egg yolks and mix well.
11. Pour the mixture into the ramekins.
12. Place the ramekins inside a small baking dish. Pour enough water in the baking dish to reach about halfway up the ramekins.
13. Bake for approximately 45 minutes.
14. Remove the dish from the oven and allow it to cool for 10 minutes for the dessert to set.

Nutritional Information
Calories 369.8, Total Fat 37.6 g,
Total Carbs 4.7 g, Approx. Net Carbs 4.7 g, Dietary Fiber 0.0 g,
Sugars 1.6 g, Protein 4.7 g

Orange Vanilla Soufflés

Serves: 4

Ingredients:
2 eggs, separated
1 cup ricotta cheese
¼ cup erythritol
1 tablespoon orange zest
1 tablespoon orange juice
1 vanilla bean, scraped
1 tablespoon chia seeds

Directions:
1. Preheat the oven to 350°F and lightly oil four ramekins.
2. Place the egg whites in a bowl and beat on high with an electric mixture until frothy.
3. Add approximately one-half of the erythritol and continue beating until stiff peaks form.
4. In another bowl, combine the remaining erythritol, ricotta cheese, and egg yolks. Cream together until smooth.
5. To the egg yolk mixture, add the orange zest, orange juice, vanilla, and chia seeds. Mix well.
6. Carefully fold the egg yolk mixture into the egg white mixture.
7. Spoon the mixture into the ramekins.
8. Place the dishes in the oven and bake for 20-25 minutes.

Nutritional Information
Calories 158.0, Total Fat 11.5 g,
Total Carbs 3.3 g, Approx. Net Carbs 2.0 g, Dietary Fiber 1.3 g,
Sugars 0.3 g, Protein 10.8 g

Tangerine Lime Keto Style Panna Cotta

Serves: 8

Ingredients:
1 ½ cups cream cheese
¼ cup butter
1 teaspoon pure vanilla extract
2 ½ teaspoons (approximately one packet) unflavored gelatin
½ cup water, boiling
½ cup tangerine juice, heated
1 tablespoon lime zest
Fresh mint for garnish

Directions:
1. In a bowl, combine the cream cheese, butter, and vanilla extract. Cream them together until smooth.
2. Place the gelatin in another bowl, and add the boiling water and tangerine juice. Stir constantly for approximately 1 minute, until the gelatin is dissolved.
3. Pour the gelatin mixture into the cream cheese mixture, along with the lime zest. Mix well, using an electric mixer, until creamy.
4. Lightly oil 8 silicone baking cups.
5. Pour an equal amount of the mixture into each cup.
6. Place the cups in the refrigerator for at least 6 hours, or overnight.
7. Flip the molds over and gently remove the baking cup.
8. Garnish with fresh mint leaves before serving.

Nutritional Information
Calories 206.4, Total Fat 20.8 g,
Total Carbs 3.3 g, Approx. Net Carbs 3.3 g, Dietary Fiber 0.0 g,
Sugars 2.9 g, Protein 3.3 g

Sweet Raspberry and Herb Mousse

Serves: 6

Ingredients:
2 ½ teaspoons unflavored gelatin powder
½ cup hot lemon verbena tea
2 cups ricotta cheese
1 cup raspberries
1 tablespoon fresh mint, chopped
1 teaspoon lemon juice
½ teaspoon vanilla extract
20 drops liquid stevia
1 cup heavy cream

Directions:
1. Place the unflavored gelatin in a small bowl. Pour the hot lemon verbena tea over the gelatin and stir until dissolved. Set the dish aside and let the mixture cool completely.
2. Next, combine the ricotta cheese, raspberries, fresh mint, lemon juice, vanilla extract, and liquid stevia in a bowl. Using an electric mixer, blend until combined and creamy.
3. Take the cooled gelatin and tea mixture and add it to the ricotta mixture. Blend until combined.
4. Next, add the heavy cream and mix on high until thickened and fluffy.
5. Spoon the mixture into chilled serving glasses.

Nutritional Information
Calories 289.6, Total Fat 25.4 g,
Total Carbs 6.0 g, Approx. Net Carbs 4.6 g, Dietary Fiber 1.4 g,
Sugars 0.3 g, Protein 10.2 g

Cookies and Bars

No Bake Macadamia Bars

Serves: 6

Ingredients:
1 cup almond flour
¼ cup flax meal
¼ cup butter, melted
¼ cup sugar free maple syrup
½ teaspoon ground ginger
½ teaspoon salt
½ cup macadamia nuts, chopped
½ cup unsweetened shredded coconut

Directions:
1. Line an 8x8 baking dish with parchment paper.
2. In a bowl, combine the almond flour, flax meal, butter, maple syrup, ginger, and salt. Mix well.
3. Next, add the macadamia nuts and coconut. Fold in until combined.
4. Spread the mixture in the baking dish, patting it down to spread the mixture out evenly.
5. Cover and refrigerate at least 2-4 hours before cutting and serving.

Nutritional Information
Calories 311.9, Total Fat 29.9 g,
Total Carbs 9.9 g, Approx. Net Carbs 4.8 g, Dietary Fiber 5.1 g,
Sugars 1.6 g, Protein 5.7 g

Macaroons

Serves: 6

Ingredients:
1 egg white
¼ cup erythritol
½ teaspoon salt
½ teaspoon cinnamon
¼ cup almonds, finely ground
1 cup unsweetened, shredded coconut, toasted
¼ cup 70% or higher cocoa content chocolate, chopped

Directions:
1. Preheat the oven to 350°F and line a baking sheet with parchment paper.
2. Place the egg white in a bowl, and beat it with an electric mixer until frothy.
3. Add the erythritol, salt, and cinnamon and continue to mix.
4. Next, add the almonds, coconut, and chocolate. Mix well.
5. Place rounded spoonfuls onto the baking sheet.
6. Place the tray in the oven and bake for 15 minutes, or until golden.

Nutritional Information
Calories 119.5, Total Fat 11.1 g,
Total Carbs 5.9 g, Approx. Net Carbs 2.6 g, Dietary Fiber 3.3 g,
Sugars 1.1 g, Protein 2.8 g

5 Layer Cashew Bars

Serves: 16

Ingredients:
1 ¼ cup almond flour
¼ cup butter, well chilled
½ cup erythritol, divided
1 teaspoon cinnamon
½ teaspoon xanthan gum
½ cup granulated stevia
1 tablespoon water
½ cup heavy whipping cream
½ cup cashew butter
1 teaspoon maple extract
1 cup cashews, chopped
½ cup unsweetened, shredded coconut, toasted
½ cup butter
¼ cup dark cocoa powder
¼ cup 70% or higher dark chocolate, chopped
20 drops liquid stevia
1 teaspoon vanilla extract

Directions:
1. Preheat the oven to 350°F and line and lightly oil an 8x8 inch baking pan.
2. In a food processor, combine the almond flour, butter, erythritol, cinnamon, and xanthan gum. Pulse until a crumbly texture is achieved.
3. Place the mixture in the baking pan and press it down to evenly distribute the mixture along the bottom of the pan.
4. Place the pan in the oven and bake for 15 minutes, or until golden brown. Remove it from the oven and let it cool.

5. Combine the granulated stevia and water in a saucepan over medium heat. Cook, stirring frequently, for approximately 5 minutes or until the mixture bubbles.
6. Remove the pan from the heat and stir in the heavy whipping cream. Return the pan to the heat and to a boil for 1-2 minutes.
7. Remove the pan from the heat again, and add the cashew butter and maple extract.
8. Spread the mixture over the baked crust layer.
9. Sprinkle the cashews on top, and then the toasted coconut. Set the pan aside to cool completely.
10. Next, combine the butter and dark cocoa powder in a saucepan over low heat. Cook for 1-2 minutes.
11. Remove the mixture from the heat and add in the chocolate, liquid stevia, and vanilla extract. Mix well until all of the chocolate is melted.
12. Drizzle the chocolate over the bars.
13. Leave the pan at room temperature until all the layers have completely set, approximately 1-2 hours.
14. Cut into squares and serve.

Nutritional Information
Calories 231.9, Total Fat 21.6 g,
Total Carbs 8.1 g, Approx. Net Carbs 5.9 g, Dietary Fiber 2.2 g,
Sugars 1.3 g, Protein 4.6 g

Chocolate Maple Bacon Cookies

Serves: 12

Ingredients:
1 ½ cups almond flour
½ cup erythritol
1 teaspoon baking powder
½ cup butter, at room temperature
1 egg
1 teaspoon maple extract
½ teaspoon vanilla extract
½ cup 70% cocoa or higher dark chocolate, chopped
1 cup bacon, cooked and crumbled

Directions:
1. In a bowl, combine the almond flour, erythritol, and baking powder. Mix well.
2. In a separate bowl cream together the butter, egg, maple extract, and vanilla extract.
3. Add the dry ingredients to the creamed butter and mix well.
4. Fold in the chocolate and the bacon.
5. Lay out a piece of plastic wrap.
6. Form the dough into a thin log and wrap it tightly with the plastic wrap. Place the log in the refrigerator to chill for at least 2 hours.
7. Preheat the oven to 325°F and line a baking sheet with parchment paper.
8. Remove the log from the refrigerator and slice it into approximately 24 pieces.
9. Place the cookies on the baking sheet and bake for 10-12 minutes, or until golden brown.

Nutritional Information
Calories 166.7, Total Fat 15.7 g,
Total Carbs 3.9 g, Approx. Net Carbs 2.3 g, Dietary Fiber 1.6 g,
Sugars 1.6 g, Protein 3.8 g

Almond Pumpkin Seed Bars

Serves: 8

Ingredients:
1 cup almond flour
½ cup butter, melted and divided
¼ cup erythritol, divided
½ teaspoon salt
¼ cup almond butter
¼ cup heavy cream
½ teaspoon cinnamon
1 teaspoon maple extract
¼ teaspoon xanthan gum
½ cup pumpkin seeds, toasted and lightly salted

Directions:
1. Preheat the oven to 400°F and line an 8x8 inch baking pan with parchment paper.
2. In a bowl, combine the almond flour, ¼ cup of the melted butter, 1 tablespoon of the erythritol, and the salt. Mix well.
3. Press the crust mixture into the bottom of the baking dish. Place it in the oven and bake for 12-15 minutes, or until browned. Remove it from the oven and let it cool.
4. In a blender, combine the remaining butter, almond butter, heavy cream, cinnamon, maple extract, and xanthan gum. Blend until creamy.
5. Spread the mixture out over the cooled crust.
6. Top with the toasted pumpkin seeds.
7. Place it in the refrigerator and let it chill for at least 2 hours or overnight.
8. Cut it into squares before serving.

Nutritional Information

Calories 261.5, Total Fat 25.2 g,
Total Carbs 6.6 g, Approx. Net Carbs 3.8 g, Dietary Fiber 2.8 g,
Sugars 0.8 g, Protein 4.7 g

Tart Lemon Lime Bars

Serves: 16

Ingredients:
1 ½ cups almond flour
½ cup unsweetened, shredded coconut
1 cup butter, melted and divided
¼ cup erythritol
1 tablespoon ginger, freshly grated
¼ cup fresh lemon juice
¼ cup fresh lime juice
1 tablespoon lime zest
6 egg yolks
½ teaspoon xanthan gum
2 tablespoons plain gelatin
¼ cup coconut for garnish, toasted and shredded
1 tablespoon fresh mint, chopped

Directions:
1. Preheat the oven to 350°F and line an 8x8 inch baking pan with parchment paper.
2. In a bowl, combine the almond flour, ½ cup coconut, ½ cup melted butter, erythritol, and ginger. Mix well.
3. Press the mixture into the bottom of the baking dish.
4. Place the baking dish in the oven and bake for 10-12 minutes, or until the crust is golden and firm.
5. Remove it from the oven and let it cool completely.
6. Place the remaining butter in a saucepan over low heat.
7. Add the lemon juice, lime juice, and lime zest. Mix well.
8. One by one, add the egg yolks, whisking quickly to incorporate them, and continue cooking while stirring until the mixture begins to thicken.
9. Remove the pan from the heat and add the xanthan gum and gelatin. Stir until dissolved.

10. Pour the mixture over the cooked crust and return the pan to the oven. Bake for 15-18 minutes, or until the bars are set in the middle.
11. Remove the pan from the oven and let it cool slightly before garnishing with toasted coconut and fresh mint.
12. Cut into bars before serving.

Nutritional Information
Calories 192.3, Total Fat 19.2 g,
Total Carbs 3.5 g, Approx. Net Carbs 2.0 g, Dietary Fiber 1.5 g,
Sugars 0.7 g, Protein 3.2 g

Dessert Bombs

Mexican Hot Chocolate Bombs

Serves: 12

Ingredients:
4 ounces cocoa butter
¼ cup unsweetened, dark cocoa powder
1 teaspoon cinnamon
½ teaspoon cayenne powder
½ teaspoon salt
¼ cup erythritol
½ cup pecans, chopped
½ cup heavy cream

Directions:
1. Line 12 mini muffin tins with cupcake liners.
2. Melt the cocoa butter to a liquid consistency in a double boiler over medium-low heat.
3. Add the cocoa powder, cinnamon, cayenne powder, and salt. Mix well.
4. Stir in the erythritol, pecans, and heavy cream. Continue cooking over medium-low heat until the mixture warms and thickens slightly.
5. Remove it from the heat and carefully pour the mixture into the prepared tins.
6. Place the tins in the freezer and freeze for at least 4 hours or overnight.
7. They can be kept in the refrigerator, for a softer texture, or in the freezer for a firmer texture, until ready to serve.

Nutritional Information
Calories 151.3, Total Fat 16.4 g,
Total Carbs 1.7 g, Approx. Net Carbs 0.7 g, Dietary Fiber 1.0 g,
Sugars 0.2 g, Protein 0.9 g

Mocha Bombs

Serves: 8

Ingredients:
1 cup mascarpone cheese
¼ cup butter
¼ cup erythritol
10 drops liquid stevia
2 tablespoons unsweetened, dark cocoa powder
¼ cup brewed espresso
½ teaspoon nutmeg

Directions:
1. Line 8 mini muffin tins with cupcake liners.
2. In a blender, combine the mascarpone cheese, butter, erythritol, stevia, and cocoa powder. Cream them together.
3. Next add the espresso and nutmeg. Blend until creamy.
4. Spoon the mixture into the prepared tins.
5. Place in the freezer for at least 4 hours before serving.

Nutritional Information
Calories 173.5, Total Fat 17.9 g,
Total Carbs 0.8 g, Approx. Net Carbs 0.3 g, Dietary Fiber 0.5 g,
Sugars 0.0 g, Protein 2.3 g

Cashew Butter Bombs

Serves: 8

Ingredients:
¼ cup cashew butter
½ cup coconut oil, melted
10 drops liquid stevia
1 teaspoon cinnamon
½ teaspoon ground ginger
1 teaspoon vanilla extract

Directions:
1. Line 8 mini muffin tins with cupcake liners.
2. Place all the ingredients in a saucepan and melt, while stirring, over low heat, just until the cashew butter softens and is easy to mix.
3. Spoon the mixture into each of the mini muffin tins.
4. Place the tin in the freezer for at least 4 hours before serving.

Nutritional Information
Calories 164.4, Total Fat 17.6 g,
Total Carbs 2.2 g, Approx. Net Carbs 2.0 g, Dietary Fiber 0.2 g,
Sugars 0.0 g, Protein 1.4 g

Lemon Lime Bombs

Serves: 12

Ingredients:
½ cup cream cheese
½ cup coconut oil
¼ cup powdered erythritol
2 cups full fat coconut milk
1 vanilla bean, scraped
1 ½ tablespoons lemon juice
1 ½ tablespoons lime juice
1 teaspoon lemon zest
1 teaspoon lime zest
Toasted unsweetened shredded coconut for topping, optional

Directions:
1. Line 12 mini muffin tins with cupcake liners.
2. Place the cream cheese, coconut oil and powdered erythritol in a bowl. Cream them together using an electric mixer.
3. Add the coconut milk, vanilla, lemon juice, lime juice, lemon zest, and lime zest. Mix until well blended.
4. Spoon the mixture into each of the muffin tins.
5. Garnish with toasted coconut, if desired.
6. Place in the freezer for at least 4 hours before serving.

Nutritional Information
Calories 119.5, Total Fat 13.2 g,
Total Carbs 0.9 g, Approx. Net Carbs 0.7 g, Dietary Fiber 0.2 g,
Sugars 0.4 g, Protein 0.7 g

Peachy Pecan Bombs

Serves: 12

Ingredients:
1 ½ cups cream cheese, softened
½ cup heavy cream
¼ cup coconut oil
¼ cup powdered erythritol
1 teaspoon vanilla extract
2 teaspoons orange zest
1 cup frozen peach slices
1 cup pecans, chopped

Directions:
1. Line 12 mini muffin tins with cupcake liners.
2. Place the cream cheese, heavy cream, coconut oil, and powdered erythritol in a blender, and blend until the ingredients are creamed together.
3. Add the vanilla extract, orange zest, peaches, and pecans. Blend until the peaches are incorporated throughout, with some chunks still remaining.
4. Spoon the mixture into the muffin tins.
5. Place in the freezer for at least 4 hours before serving.

Nutritional Information
Calories 247.2, Total Fat 25.4 g,
Total Carbs 4.4 g, Approx. Net Carbs 3.2 g, Dietary Fiber 1.2 g,
Sugars 2.6 g, Protein 3.4 g

Double Berry Mint Bombs

Serves: 12

Ingredients:
½ cup cream cheese, softened
½ cup ricotta cheese
½ cup heavy cream
¼ cup coconut oil
¼ cup powdered erythritol
1 teaspoon vanilla extract
1 tablespoon lemon juice
½ cup blueberries
½ cup raspberries
¼ cup fresh mint, chopped

Directions:
1. Line 12 mini muffin tins with cupcake liners.
2. Place the cream cheese, ricotta cheese, heavy cream, coconut oil, and erythritol in a bowl.
3. Using an electric mixer, cream the ingredients together.
4. Add the vanilla extract, lemon juice, blueberries, and raspberries.
5. Blend again, using the electric mixer, until the mixture is creamy and the berries are broken up and blended in.
6. Stir in the mint.
7. Spoon the mixture into the muffin tins.
8. Place them in the freezer for at least 4 hours before serving.

Nutritional Information
Calories 126.5, Total Fat 12.4 g,
Total Carbs 2.6 g, Approx. Net Carbs 2.1 g, Dietary Fiber 0.5 g,
Sugars 1.0 g, Protein 2.2 g

Sweet and Savory Chocolate Bombs

Serves: 12

Ingredients:
1 ½ cups mascarpone cheese
¼ cup heavy cream
¼ cup powdered erythritol
¼ cup brewed espresso
1 teaspoon vanilla extract
1 teaspoon cinnamon
1 tablespoon dark cocoa powder
2 teaspoons orange zest
¼ cup cooked bacon, crumbled

Directions:
1. Line 12 mini muffin tins with cupcake liners.
2. Place the mascarpone cheese, heavy cream, and erythritol in a bowl. Using an electric mixer, cream them together.
3. Add the espresso, vanilla extract, cinnamon, dark cocoa powder, and orange zest. Blend well.
4. Stir in the crumbled bacon.
5. Spoon the mixture into each of the muffin tins.
6. Place them in the freezer for at least 4 hours before serving.

Nutritional Information
Calories 142.9, Total Fat 14.3 g,
Total Carbs 0.4 g, Approx. Net Carbs 0.2 g, Dietary Fiber 0.2 g,
Sugars 0.0 g, Protein 0.5 g

Maple Pecan Bombs

Serves: 12

Ingredients:
½ cup mascarpone cheese
½ cup almond butter
¼ cup butter
¼ cup powdered erythritol
1 tablespoon rum
2 teaspoons maple extract
½ cup pecans, chopped

Directions:
1. Line 12 mini muffin tins with cupcake liners.
2. Place the mascarpone cheese, almond butter, butter, powdered erythritol, rum, and maple extract in a bowl.
3. Using an electric mixer, blend the ingredients together until creamy.
4. Stir in the pecans.
5. Spoon the mixture into the muffin tins.
6. Place them in the freezer for at least 4 hours before serving.

Nutritional Information
Calories 192.0, Total Fat 19.2 g,
Total Carbs 2.9 g, Approx. Net Carbs 1.4 g, Dietary Fiber 1.5 g,
Sugars 0.7 g, Protein 2.1 g

Coconut Mint Bombs

Serves: 12

Ingredients:
1 ½ cups mascarpone cheese
¼ cup coconut oil
¼ cup powdered erythritol
1 teaspoon vanilla extract
½ cup unsweetened shredded coconut
¼ cup fresh mint, chopped

Directions:
1. Line 12 mini muffin tins with cupcake liners.
2. Place the mascarpone cheese, coconut oil, powdered erythritol, and vanilla extract in a bowl.
3. Using an electric mixer, blend the ingredients together until creamy.
4. Stir in the coconut and fresh mint.
5. Spoon the mixture into each of the muffin tins.
6. Place them in the freezer for at least 4 hours before serving.

Nutritional Information
Calories 181.4, Total Fat 18.8 g,
Total Carbs 0.9 g, Approx. Net Carbs 0.5 g, Dietary Fiber 0.4 g,
Sugars 0.2 g, Protein 0.2 g

Ketolicious Mug Cakes

Vanilla Bean Mug Cake

Serves: 1

Ingredients:
3 tablespoons almond flour
⅛ teaspoon baking soda
2 tablespoons erythritol
1 egg
1 vanilla bean, scraped
½ teaspoon vanilla extract
½ teaspoon nutmeg
1 tablespoon coconut oil, melted

Directions:
1. Preheat the oven to 350°F and lightly oil an ovenproof mug or ramekin.
2. Combine the almond flour, baking soda, and erythritol together in the mug.
3. Add the egg and whisk until blended.
4. Next, add the vanilla bean, vanilla extract, nutmeg, and coconut oil. Mix well.
5. Place the mug or ramekin in the oven and bake for 20 minutes, or until the cake is golden brown.

Nutritional Information
Calories 325.8, Total Fat 30.1 g,
Total Carbs 5.5 g, Approx. Net Carbs 2.6 g, Dietary Fiber 2.9 g,
Sugars 1.1 g, Protein 11.3 g

Spiced Mug Cake

Serves: 1

Ingredients:
2 tablespoons almond flour
1 tablespoon coconut flour
2 tablespoons erythritol
⅛ teaspoon baking soda
1 egg
1 teaspoon cinnamon
½ teaspoon nutmeg
½ teaspoon ground ginger
1 tablespoon cream cheese
1 tablespoon coconut milk
5 drops liquid stevia

Directions:
1. Preheat the oven to 350°F and lightly oil an ovenproof mug or ramekin.
2. Combine the almond flour, coconut flour, erythritol, and baking soda in the mug.
3. Add the egg and whisk until blended.
4. Next, add the cinnamon, nutmeg, and ground ginger. Mix well.
5. Place the mug or ramekin in the oven and bake for 20 minutes, or until it is golden brown.
6. While the mug cake is cooking, combine the cream cheese, coconut milk, and liquid stevia. Mix until creamy.
7. Once the mug cake has cooled, spread the cream cheese frosting over the top, and enjoy.

Nutritional Information
Calories 260.9, Total Fat 21.8 g,
Total Carbs 6.2 g, Approx. Net Carbs 3.2 g, Dietary Fiber 3.0 g,
Sugars 1.6 g, Protein 12.4 g

Ultimate Cocoa Mug Cake

Serves: 1

Ingredients:
2 tablespoons almond flour
1 tablespoon coconut flour
¼ teaspoon baking powder
2 tablespoons erythritol
1 egg
2 tablespoons butter, melted
2 tablespoons unsweetened dark cocoa powder
1 teaspoon espresso powder
½ teaspoon cinnamon
½ teaspoon vanilla extract
Sugar free whipped topping for garnish (optional)

Directions:
1. Preheat the oven to 350°F and lightly oil an ovenproof mug or ramekin.
2. Combine the almond flour, coconut flour, baking powder, and erythritol together in the mug.
3. Add the egg and whisk until blended.
4. Next, add the melted butter, unsweetened dark cocoa powder, espresso powder, cinnamon, and vanilla extract. Mix well.
5. Place the mug or ramekin in the oven and bake for 20 minutes, or until it is set in the center.
6. Let it cool, and garnish with whipped topping, if desired.

Nutritional Information
Calories 432.6, Total Fat 40.5 g,
Total Carbs 11.5 g, Approx. Net Carbs 4.6 g, Dietary Fiber 6.9 g,
Sugars 1.1 g, Protein 13.5 g

Blackberries and Cream Mug Cake

Serves: 1

Ingredients:
2 tablespoons almond flour
1 tablespoon coconut flour
⅛ teaspoon baking soda
2 tablespoons erythritol
1 egg
1 tablespoon butter, melted
1 tablespoon unsweetened, shredded coconut
½ teaspoon vanilla extract
½ teaspoon ground ginger
¼ cup blackberries
1 tablespoon heavy whipping cream

Directions:
1. Preheat the oven to 350°F and lightly oil an ovenproof mug or ramekin.
2. Combine the almond flour, coconut flour, baking soda, and erythritol together in a mug.
3. Add the egg and whisk until combined.
4. Next, add the melted butter, unsweetened shredded coconut, vanilla extract, and ground ginger. Mix well.
5. Stir in the blackberries.
6. Place the mug or ramekin in the oven and bake for 20 minutes, or until the cake is golden brown.
7. Let it cool slightly and pour the heavy cream over the top just before serving.

Nutritional Information
Calories 414.4, Total Fat 37.1 g,
Total Carbs 11.9 g, Approx. Net Carbs 6.4 g, Dietary Fiber 5.5 g,
Sugars 4.0 g, Protein 12.3 g

Chocolate Bacon Mug Cake

Serves: 1

Ingredients:
3 tablespoons almond flour
⅛ teaspoon baking soda
2 tablespoons erythritol
1 egg
1 tablespoon butter, melted
½ teaspoon cinnamon
1 teaspoon orange juice
1 tablespoon unsweetened dark cocoa powder
1 tablespoon cooked bacon, crumbled
1 tablespoon walnuts, chopped

Directions:
1. Preheat the oven to 350°F and lightly oil an ovenproof mug or ramekin.
2. Combine the almond flour, baking soda, and erythritol in a mug.
3. Add the egg, and whisk until blended.
4. Next, add the butter, cinnamon, orange juice, and cocoa powder. Mix well.
5. Stir in the bacon and walnuts.
6. Place the mug or ramekin in the oven and bake for 20 minutes, or until it is set in the middle.

Nutritional Information
Calories 397.5, Total Fat 35.6 g,
Total Carbs 10.5 g, Approx.Net Carbs 4.6 g, Dietary Fiber 5.9 g,
Sugars 1.3 g, Protein 14.5 g

Peanut Butter Cookie Mug Cake

Serves: 1

Ingredients:
2 tablespoons coconut flour
¼ teaspoon baking powder
1 egg
1 tablespoon butter, melted
2 tablespoons sugar free peanut butter
1 tablespoon almond milk
½ teaspoon maple extract
½ teaspoon vanilla extract
1 tablespoon peanuts, chopped
Whipped coconut cream, optional

Directions:
1. Preheat the oven to 350°F and lightly oil an ovenproof mug or ramekin.
2. Combine the coconut flour and baking powder in the mug.
3. Add the egg and whisk until blended.
4. Next, add the melted butter, sugar free peanut butter, almond milk, maple extract, and vanilla extract. Mix well.
5. Stir in the peanuts.
6. Place the mug or ramekin in the oven and bake for 20 minutes, or until the cake is golden brown.
7. Allow it to cool slightly and top with whipped coconut cream, if desired.

Nutritional Information
Calories 363.7, Total Fat 32.5 g,
Total Carbs 7.5 g, Approx. Net Carbs 3.8 g, Dietary Fiber 3.7 g,
Sugars 1.5 g, Protein 13.6 g

Elegant Pies

Mini PB&J Pies

Serves: 4

Ingredients:
¼ cup almond flour
¼ cup flaxseed meal
1 egg white
1 tablespoon erythritol
¼ cup natural peanut butter
1 avocado, cubed
¼ cup heavy cream
1 teaspoon vanilla extract
1 cup blackberries
½ cup cream cheese
¼ cup peanuts, finely chopped

Directions:
1. Preheat the oven to 350°F and lightly oil four mini pie or tart tins.
2. In a blender, combine the almond flour, flaxseed meal, egg white, and erythritol. Mix until crumbly but formable.
3. Press the crust mixture into each of the prepared mini tins.
4. Place the tins in the oven and bake for 10 minutes, then remove them and allow them to cool.
5. In the blender, combine the peanut butter, avocado, heavy cream, and vanilla extract. Blend until creamy.
6. Spread the mixture evenly into each of the prepared crusts.
7. Place the pies in the refrigerator and chill for 30 minutes.

8. While the pies are chilling, combine the blackberries and cream cheese in a blender. Add a little heavy cream if needed to thin the mixture out into a thick, but spreadable, consistency.
9. Remove the pies from the refrigerator and spread the blackberry mixture over each.
10. Garnish with chopped peanuts.
11. Place the pies in the refrigerator and chill an additional 30 minutes before serving.

Nutritional Information
Calories 473.2, Total Fat 40.1 g,
Total Carbs 18.2 g, Approx.Net Carbs 8.9 g, Dietary Fiber 9.3 g,
Sugars 4.7 g, Protein 13.4 g

Creamy Lime Pie

Serves: 8

Ingredients:
1 ½ cups almond flour
½ cup erythritol, divided
½ teaspoon salt
¼ cup butter, melted
1 cup heavy cream
4 egg yolks
⅓ cup freshly squeezed key lime juice
1 tablespoon lime zest
¼ cup cold butter, cubed
1 teaspoon vanilla extract
¼ teaspoon xanthan gum
1 cup sour cream
½ cup cream cheese

Directions:
1. Preheat the oven to 350°F.
2. In a bowl, combine the almond flour, ¼ cup of the erythritol, and salt.
3. Slowly add the melted butter to the mixture, and blend.
4. Press the mixture evenly into a pie dish.
5. Place the pie dish in the oven and bake for approximately 15 minutes, or until the crust is lightly browned. Remove it from the oven and allow it to cool.
6. In a saucepan, combine the heavy cream, egg yolks, remaining erythritol, lime juice and lime zest. Heat over medium, using a whisk to stir frequently, until the mixture begins to thicken, approximately 7-10 minutes.
7. Remove the saucepan from the heat and add the cold butter, vanilla extract, xanthan gum, sour cream, and cream cheese. Whisk until it is smooth and creamy.

8. Transfer the mixture into the pie shell.
9. Cover and refrigerate for at least 4 hours or overnight.

Nutritional Information
Calories 386.4, Total Fat 38.6 g,
Total Carbs 6.4 g, Approx. Net Carbs 4.2 g, Dietary Fiber 2.2 g,
Sugars 1.4 g, Protein 7.0 g

Luscious and Fluffy Lemon Pie

Serves: 8

Ingredients:
½ cup powdered erythritol
1 tablespoon arrowroot powder
1 cup fresh lemon juice
4 whole eggs plus 4 egg yolks
1 tablespoon lemon zest
1 teaspoon vanilla extract
½ cup butter, cubed
1 cup almond flour
½ cup unsweetened shredded coconut
¼ cup erythritol
½ teaspoon salt
¼ cup butter, melted
1 ½ cups heavy whipping cream
2 tablespoons erythritol
1 teaspoon vanilla extract
¼ teaspoon xanthan gum

Directions:
1. Place the powdered erythritol and arrowroot powder together in a saucepan and mix until combined.
2. Add the lemon juice, whole eggs, and egg yolks. Whisk them together until they are blended.
3. Place the saucepan over medium heat and add the lemon zest and vanilla. Whisk constantly until the mixture begins to thicken.
4. Once the mixture thickens, reduce the heat to low and continue whisking for 1-2 additional minutes.
5. Remove the saucepan from the heat and add the cubed butter. Whisk until well combined.

6. Pour the mixture into a clean container, cover tightly with plastic wrap, and chill for at least 4 hours.
7. While the lemon filling is chilling, preheat the oven to 350°F.
8. In a bowl, combine the almond flour, unsweetened shredded coconut, ¼ cup erythritol, salt, and melted butter. Mix until crumbly.
9. Press the mixture into a 9-inch pie dish.
10. Place it in the oven and bake for 10-12 minutes, or until it is golden brown, then remove it from the oven and let it cool completely.
11. When you are ready to assemble the pie, combine the whipping cream, 2 tablespoons erythritol, vanilla extract, and xanthan gum in a medium-sized mixing bowl.
12. Using an electric mixer, blend until it is thick with firm peaks.
13. Remove the lemon filling from the refrigerator and transfer it to a bowl.
14. Add ¼ of the whipped topping to the lemon filling, and beat it with an electric mixer.
15. Reserve about half of the remaining whipped cream for the top of the pie and add the rest to the lemon filling. Stir until thoroughly combined.
16. Spoon the filling into the prepared pie crust and spread it evenly. Smooth the top.
17. Pipe the remaining whipped cream over the top.
18. Chill the pie in the refrigerator for at least 2 hours before serving.

Nutritional Information
Calories 483.0, Total Fat 47.6 g,
Total Carbs 9.1 g, Approx. Net Carbs 6.8 g, Dietary Fiber 2.3 g,
Sugars 1.7 g, Protein 8.5 g

Coconut Chocolate Layered Pie

Serves: 8

Ingredients:
2 cups almond flour
2 cups unsweetened shredded coconut, divided
¼ cup erythritol
1 teaspoon cinnamon
½ cup butter, melted
1 cup cream cheese
½ cup powdered erythritol, divided
¼ cup full fat coconut milk
1 teaspoon coconut extract
2 cups heavy cream
2 tablespoons unsweetened dark cocoa powder
1 teaspoon vanilla extract
1 tablespoon rum or 1 teaspoon rum extract
Dark chocolate shavings for garnish (optional)

Directions:
1. Preheat the oven to 350°F.
2. In a bowl, combine the almond flour, 1 cup of the unsweetened shredded coconut, ¼ cup erythritol, cinnamon, and butter. Mix them together until crumbly.
3. Press the mixture into a 9-inch pie dish.
4. Place the crust in the oven and bake for 10-12 minutes, or until it is golden. Remove it from the oven and let it cool completely.
5. Combine the cream cheese, ¼ cup powdered erythritol, coconut milk, coconut extract and the remaining unsweetened, shredded coconut.
6. Using an electric mixer, blend the ingredients together until they are smooth and creamy.
7. Spread the mixture in the prepared pie crust.

8. In another bowl, combine the heavy cream, dark cocoa powder, remaining erythritol, vanilla extract, and rum or rum extract. Mix on high until thickened with peaks forming.
9. Spoon the mixture over the coconut layer in the pie dish and smooth it out to create an even surface.
10. Garnish with shaved chocolate, if desired.
11. Place the pie in the refrigerator for at least 4 hours or overnight before serving.

Nutritional Information
Calories 680.2, Total Fat 68.9 g,
Total Carbs 14.1 g, Approx. Net Carbs 8.0 g, Dietary Fiber 6.1 g,
Sugars 3.3 g, Protein 10.1 g

Spiced Ricotta Pie

Serves: 8

Ingredients:
1 ½ cups almond flour
½ cup unsweetened, shredded coconut
½ teaspoon salt
¼ cup butter, melted
4 eggs
1 vanilla bean, scraped
2 cups ricotta cheese
1 tablespoon coconut powder
1 teaspoon cinnamon
½ teaspoon nutmeg
2 teaspoons lemon juice
1 cup erythritol

Directions:
1. Preheat the oven to 350°F.
2. In a bowl, combine the almond flour, unsweetened shredded coconut, salt, and melted butter. Mix until crumbly.
3. Press the mixture into a 9-inch pie dish, and bake it for 10-12 minutes, or until it is golden brown.
4. Remove the pie crust from the oven and allow it to cool slightly.
5. Place the eggs and vanilla in a bowl and beat them until they are frothy.
6. Add the ricotta cheese, coconut powder, cinnamon, nutmeg, lemon juice, and erythritol. Mix until blended and creamy.
7. Spoon the mixture into the prepared pie crust.
8. Place the pie in the oven and bake for 40-45 minutes, or until it is lightly browned and set in the center.

Nutritional Information

Calories 329.7, Total Fat 28.3 g,
Total Carbs 7.2 g, Approx. Net Carbs 4.3 g, Dietary Fiber 2.9 g,
Sugars 1.3 g, Protein 14.2 g

Crustless Strawberry Custard Pie

Serves: 8

Ingredients:
3 eggs
2 cups heavy whipping cream
½ cup erythritol
1 teaspoon vanilla
1 cup strawberries, chopped
1 teaspoon ground ginger
½ teaspoon cinnamon
¼ teaspoon salt

Directions:
1. Preheat the oven to 425°F and lightly oil a 9-inch pie dish.
2. Place the eggs in a bowl and whisk until they are foamy.
3. Add the heavy whipping cream, erythritol, and vanilla. Mix well.
4. Sprinkle the strawberries with ground ginger, cinnamon, and salt.
5. Spread the strawberries in the bottom of the pie dish.
6. Pour the custard over the strawberries.
7. Place the pie dish in the oven and bake for 10 minutes.
8. Reduce the heat to 325°F and bake for an additional 30 minutes, or until golden and set in the center.
9. Let cool before serving.

Nutritional Information
Calories 238.0, Total Fat 23.9 g,
Total Carbs 3.1 g, Approx. Net Carbs 2.7 g, Dietary Fiber 0.4 g,
Sugars 1.1 g, Protein 3.7 g

Rich and Silky Ice Creams
Sweet Raspberries and Cream Ice Cream

Serves: 6

Ingredients:
1 cup heavy cream
¼ cup erythritol
3 egg yolks
½ cup mascarpone cheese
1 teaspoon vanilla extract
1 tablespoon lemon juice
1 teaspoon lemon zest
1 cup raspberries

Directions:
1. Place the heavy cream and erythritol in a saucepan and warm over medium heat, stirring frequently until the erythritol is dissolved. Remove the saucepan from the heat.
2. Place the egg yolks in a bowl and slowly add approximately ¼ cup of the warm cream mixture, whisking the entire time, to temper the eggs.
3. Slowly add the rest of the cream mixture to the eggs while whisking constantly.
4. Next, add the mascarpone cheese, vanilla extract, lemon juice, and lemon zest. Stir until well combined.
5. Fold in the raspberries.
6. Pour the mixture into an ice cream maker and follow the manufacturer's directions.
7. Serve in well chilled glasses.

Nutritional Information
Calories 254.4, Total Fat 25.0 g,
Total Carbs 3.8 g, Approx. Net Carbs 2.4 g, Dietary Fiber 1.4 g,
Sugars 0.1 g, Protein 2.3 g

Blueberry Pistachio Ice Cream

Serves: 8

Ingredients:
1 cup full fat coconut milk
1 cup heavy cream
¼ cup erythritol
½ cup cashew butter
1 cup ricotta cheese
1 teaspoon vanilla extract
¼ teaspoon xanthan gum
1 cup blueberries
½ cup pistachios, chopped

Directions:
1. Place the coconut milk and heavy cream in a saucepan over medium heat and stir frequently.
2. Once the liquid is heated through and steaming, add the erythritol and stir until it is dissolved.
3. Remove the pan from the heat.
4. Pour the mixture into a container that can be used with an immersion blender.
5. Add the cashew butter, ricotta cheese, vanilla extract, and xanthan gum.
6. Blend until creamy.
7. Transfer the mixture to a bowl, and fold in the blueberries and pistachios.
8. Pour it into an ice cream maker, and follow the manufacturer's directions.
9. Serve in well chilled glasses.

Nutritional Information
Calories 285.2, Total Fat 24.9 g,
Total Carbs 10.0 g, Approx.Net Carbs 8.4 g, Dietary Fiber 1.6 g,
Sugars 2.6 g, Protein 7.9 g

Pumpkin Butter Pecan Ice Cream

Serves: 6

Ingredients:
¼ cup butter
1 cup pecans, chopped
½ teaspoon salt
½ teaspoon cinnamon
½ cup mascarpone cheese
½ cup cooked pumpkin, mashed
1 teaspoon ground ginger
½ teaspoon coriander
3 pasteurized egg yolks
1 ½ cups heavy cream
2 teaspoons maple extract
½ teaspoon xanthan gum
20 drops liquid stevia

Directions:
1. Place the butter in a skillet and melt it over medium heat.
2. Add the pecans, and season them with salt and cinnamon. Cook, stirring frequently, for approximately 5 minutes, or until the pecans are toasted.
3. Place the mascarpone cheese, pumpkin, ground ginger, coriander, egg yolks, heavy cream, maple extract, xanthan gum, and liquid stevia in a blender. Blend until smooth and creamy.
4. Pour the mixture into a bowl. Add the pecans and any remaining butter from the pan. Stir well.
5. Transfer the mixture to an ice cream maker and follow the manufacturer's directions.
6. Serve in well chilled glasses.

Nutritional Information

Calories 329.5, Total Fat 33.6 g,
Total Carbs 4.2 g, Approx. Net Carbs 2.1 g, Dietary Fiber 2.1 g,
Sugars 1.0 g, Protein 3.5 g

Triple Nut Vanilla Ice cream

Serves: 6

Ingredients:
1 cup heavy whipping cream
¼ cup erythritol
3 egg yolks
¼ cup butter, softened
¼ cup plain yogurt
2 vanilla beans, scraped
1 teaspoon vanilla extract
1 teaspoon walnut extract
½ teaspoon salt
¼ cup walnuts, chopped
¼ cup pecans, chopped
¼ cup cashews, chopped

Directions:
1. Combine the heavy cream and erythritol together in a saucepan over medium heat.
2. Stir constantly until the erythritol is dissolved. Remove the pan from the heat.
3. Place the eggs in a bowl.
4. Take approximately ¼ cup of the cream mixture and slowly pour it into the eggs, whisking constantly to temper the eggs.
5. Slowly add the remaining cream to the eggs, whisking constantly.
6. Transfer the mixture to a blender and add the butter, yogurt, vanilla, vanilla extract, walnut extract, and salt. Blend until creamy.
7. Transfer the mixture back to a bowl and stir in the walnuts, pecans, and cashews.

8. Pour it into an ice cream maker, and follow the manufacturer's directions.
9. Serve in well chilled glasses.

Nutritional Information

Calories 338.2, Total Fat 34.5 g,
Total Carbs 5.1 g, Approx. Net Carbs 4.1 g, Dietary Fiber 1.0 g,
Sugars 1.2 g, Protein 4.7 g

Lemon and Almond Chia Ice Cream

Serves: 6

Ingredients:
1 cup heavy whipping cream
2 cups full fat coconut milk
¼ cup erythritol
2 egg yolks
½ cup fresh lemon juice
¼ teaspoon xanthan gum
1 teaspoon vanilla extract
1 tablespoon chia seeds
1 tablespoon lemon zest
¼ cup almonds, chopped

Directions:
1. Combine the heavy whipping cream, coconut milk, and erythritol in a saucepan over medium heat.
2. Stir constantly until the erythritol is dissolved, and remove it from the heat.
3. Place the eggs in a bowl and add approximately ¼ cup of the warm cream mixture, slowly, to the eggs while whisking constantly.
4. Slowly add the remaining cream mixture to the eggs, still whisking constantly.
5. Add the lemon juice, xanthan gum, vanilla extract, chia seeds, lemon zest, and chopped almonds. Mix well.
6. Transfer the mixture to an ice cream maker and follow the manufacturer's directions.
7. Serve in well chilled glasses.

Nutritional Information

Calories 208.0, Total Fat 20.4 g,
Total Carbs 5.4 g, Approx. Net Carbs 3.7 g, Dietary Fiber 1.7 g,
Sugars 0.7 g, Protein 3.1 g

Vanilla Coconut Latte Ice Cream

Serves: 6

Ingredients:
1 cup full fat coconut milk
1 cup heavy whipping cream
25 drops liquid stevia
½ cup crème fraîche
½ cup strong brewed espresso
1 vanilla bean, scraped
1 teaspoon coconut extract
1 cup unsweetened, shredded coconut

Directions:
1. Combine the coconut milk, heavy cream, liquid stevia, crème fraîche, espresso, vanilla, and coconut extract in a blender. Blend until smooth and creamy.
2. Stir in the coconut.
3. Transfer the mixture to an ice cream maker and follow the manufacturer's directions.
4. Serve in well chilled glasses.

Nutritional Information
Calories 306.6, Total Fat 31.7 g,
Total Carbs 5.7 g, Approx. Net Carbs 3.8 g, Dietary Fiber 1.9 g,
Sugars 1.6 g, Protein 2.4 g

Conclusion

Making a commitment to any diet or style of eating is a big deal. It requires forethought, research and diligence. You are hoping to gain something from eating the ketogenic way, and you will – as long as you make ketogenic eating a part of your lifestyle. That said, it can be difficult to adopt something as a long term lifestyle change if you feel that something is missing, in this case dessert. Ketogenic diets, or any low carb eating plan for that matter, are notorious for the savory decadence that you are allowed, however little attention is really given to how you will satisfy your sweet tooth. If you have ever tried a diet in the past, then you know that sometimes the road to quitting is paved with cravings. Here, with this book, the goal has been to show you that you can have your ketogenic diet and eat your sweets too. Each recipe has been crafted to suit your ketogenic needs while satisfying your sweet tooth. Whether it is just a quick sweet bite you are after, or a celebratory dessert to share with others, you don't need to sabotage your diet to fulfill your cravings. Part of life should be sweet, and sometimes you should even eat dessert first.

More Books from Madison Miller

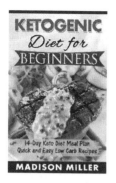 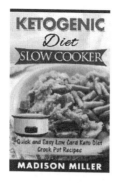 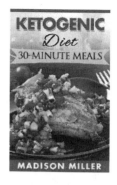

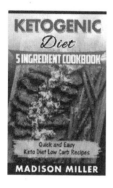 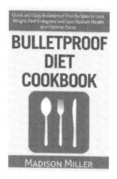 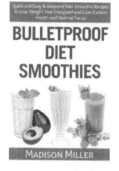

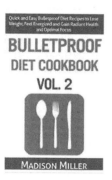 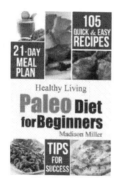 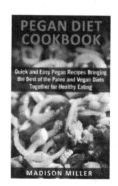

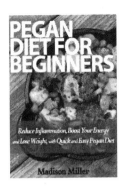

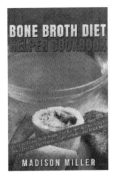

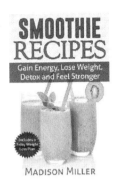

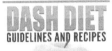

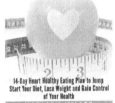

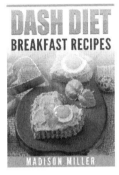

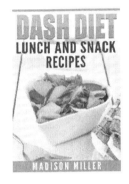

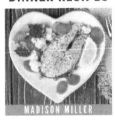

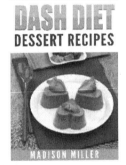

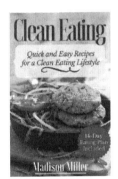

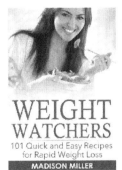

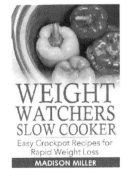

Appendix - Cooking Conversion Charts

1. Measuring Equivalent Chart

Type	Imperial	Imperial	Metric
Weight	1 dry ounce		28g
	1 pound	16 dry ounces	0.45 kg
Volume	1 teaspoon		5 ml
	1 dessert spoon	2 teaspoons	10 ml
	1 tablespoon	3 teaspoons	15 ml
	1 Australian tablespoon	4 teaspoons	20 ml
	1 fluid ounce	2 tablespoons	30 ml
	1 cup	16 tablespoons	240 ml
	1 cup	8 fluid ounces	240 ml
	1 pint	2 cups	470 ml
	1 quart	2 pints	0.95 l
	1 gallon	4 quarts	3.8 l
Length	1 inch		2.54 cm

*   Numbers are rounded to the closest equivalent

2. Oven Temperature Equivalent Chart

T(°F)	T(°C)
220	100
225	110
250	120
275	140
300	150
325	160
350	180
375	190
400	200
425	220
450	230
475	250
500	260

*   T(°C) = [T(°F)-32] * 5/9

**   T(°F) = T(°C) * 9/5 + 32

*** Numbers are rounded to the closest equivalent

Made in the USA
Lexington, KY
20 March 2018